Pain Relief Remedies:

TOP 30 Natural Recipes With Essential Oils

And Herbs To Relief Your Pain Instantly

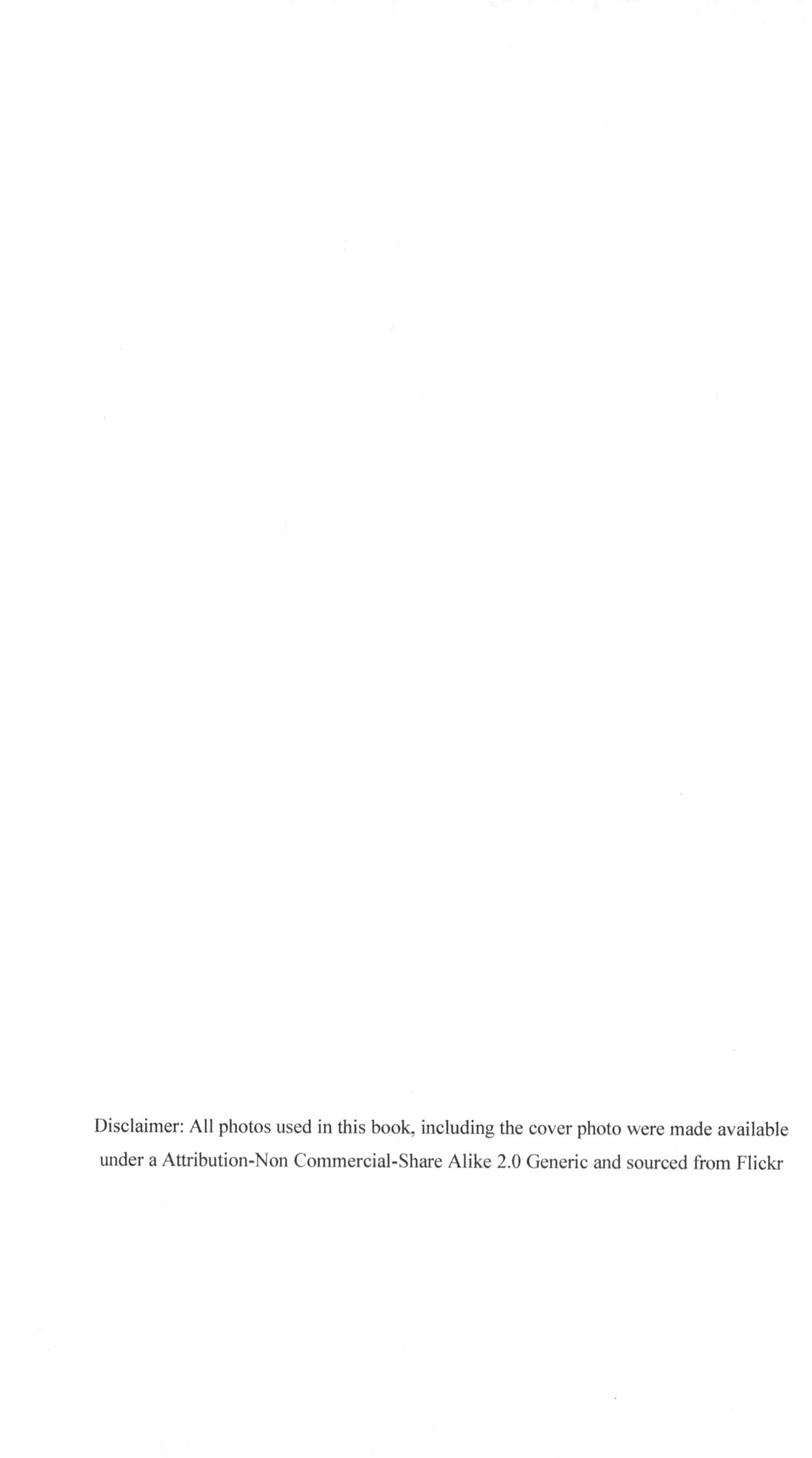

Table of content:

Introduction

Many of us suffer daily from aches and pains the technical term is 'Myalgia', which is translated to mean 'pain in the muscles.' One of these pains that is most common is called 'Fibromyalgia.' This is a very devastating disorder that involves the musculoskeletal system, followed by wide spread pain in the body that is accompanied with deep fatigue.

Some look at Fibromyalgia as the mother load of all aches and pains, it is caused by the imbalance of chemicals that causes a disruption which when the brain processes the signals it relates to them as pain signals. The good news is that there are medicinal herbs that can help treat this painful ailment and even possibly reverse it all together.

Using medicinal herbs can help to readjust and refine those pain processors of the brain, this will in turn allow you to rework how your body is interpreting external stressors. As our bodies age Fibromyalgia is just a magnification of the discomfort our bodies face the older we get. It is a deep rooted pain that is in our muscle tissue that can lead to much discomfort especially as our bodies age.

The human body is basically like a machine that with prolonged use it begins to wear out. But with some healthy herbs thrown into the mix these can really help to combat whatever it is that ails. Let us take a look at some healthy organic aids that can help you combat your aches and pains in life.

One of the most important things before picking the right herbs is to have the basic knowledge about its usage. It is really important that you identify herbs correctly. We have provided photographs of most of these herbs and have added additional information about their appearance so that you can hand-pick the natural herbs of your choice.

After when you have identified the natural products that can help you survive, the second most important factor is regarding their correct usage. We have listed the most appropriate way to use these herbs and how they can help you in various ways. A proper listing of their benefits has been provided so that you can figure out how and when to use these herbs correctly.

A single herb can be of numerous usages and you should certainly keep a few of them with you when you move, as an unforeseen disaster might come unannounced. A wide range of natural herbs have been discussed in the guide – from edible products to antiseptic ones, anti-inflammatory herbs to plants that can help in skin treatment, and more.

Using the essential oil Ylang Ylang can help in achieving balance in the hormones. Wild Orange essential oil is great at helping to purify the skin and boost the immunity system. When it comes to the benefits of essential oils it is difficult to list all of them. The reason being is that nature has a special way of producing results from unexpected places and benefits of one essential oil can cover so many aspects in life.

Take the example of wild orange essential oil, it can be used for dual or even triple purpose. It can be used to help boost the immunity system, skin and also to help protect the body from seasonal changes in the atmosphere and weather conditions. This essential oil can help to refresh the mind and leave you feeling invigorated, so you don't need to limit your use of essential oils to only when you are ill.

Use essential oils as a prevention that you can incorporate into your life. Adding essential oils into your life will help you to avoid illnesses so that you do not have to deal with the pressure of dealing with them. It is definitely a wiser choice to choose prevention rather than waiting to you are ill and need to seek a cure. Why put your body through undo stress when you do not have to.

Chapter 1. The chemical composition of medicinal herbs

There is some specific composition of medicinal herb, which makes them useful for serving the purpose as a curative. For majority of the medical issues herbs are considered useful because of the presence of any of the following chemicals or agents in the herb:

- Terpenes
- Tartaric acids
- Tannins
- Saponins
- Mucilage
- Glycosides
- Flavonoids
- Essential oils
- Coumarins
- Citric acid
- Bitter compounds
- Antibiotics
- Alkaloids

The presence of any of these elements will make sure that that the medicinal properties of herbs are ensured. A lot of medicinal herbs may contain even more than one chemical agent and thus enhancing the curative capabilities of a particular medicine. The mixture of these agents is used in pharmaceutical industry to make up various medicines.

People are getting more educated and realizing the harm that they are causing their bodies by feeding on synthetic and unnatural substances with bad side effects they are turning more and more to natural solutions to their aches and pains. Many modern treatments are becoming incredibly expensive and for many people that do not have some kind of health coverage they simply cannot afford to use modern methods of treatment.

However, with this being said we are also finding out that not only is medicinal medicine a more affordable choice for many but it is in fact considered by more and more people to be the safest and healthiest choice as a form of treatment for our various ailments.

When you sit down and really think about it what would seem to you the more healthy choice—the synthetic drug with severe side effects or the natural medicinal herbal treatment? I myself lean towards taking the natural choice as a form of treatment.

If you get the thumbs up from your physician to try the natural remedy for your ailment, then why not give it a try all you may have to lose is not suffering from nasty side effects as well as putting foreign substances into your body that are made of unnatural ingredients. This in itself should have you sitting wondering how good these foreign substances could really be for my health in the end.

You need to know that there are a few wild species of plants, which are not edible. Some of them can also be injurious to health.

So, even though the plants we will be talking about are actually helpful, you should not eat just about anything and do not use your half knowledge. You need to be sure that you are picking the right medicinal plants and you are aware of the benefits that it offers.

In addition, one plant may not offer multiple benefits and sometimes you need to be wary of a few conditions, which may be imposed on it. Only when you are aware of every single detail should you proceed with the use of herbal medicines in the world.

Without our immune system, we could not step out into the world beyond our front door, so it is very important in our survival. If we did not have it we would have to live in a bubble to protect ourselves from contaminates.

Included in your immune system is an army of white blood cells that fight against harmful bacteria and viruses on a daily basis. Your body will produce around 1000 white blood cells a day. The specialized part of your white blood cell army is called 'Macrophages' these go seek out any germs that may enter your system and once they locate them they destroy them.

We remain healthy largely due to our immune system being able to filter and eliminate harmful elements. It is good to give our immune system a little jumpstart once and a while.

Benefits of herbs

Often called as natural aspirin or the natural miracle drug, it has a wide range of benefits that can help you save your life in the wild.

- If you are out in the wild and is suffering from an extreme headache after being exposed to severe natural conditions, then you must apply some willow on your forehead. You can also consume it directly for immediate relief. It has been proven that willow has more power than general aspirin to cure a headache.

- If after walking for a long duration, you are having pain in your body, then a little intake of willow will cure it immediately. From osteoarthritis to arthritis, the magical drug can treat it all.

- After being exposed in the wild, your skin might suffer from wear and tear. You can prepare an ointment by boiling willow and apply it on your skin. It not only will act as an antiseptic, but will also cure your wounds and burns.

- Salicylate is one such substance that is present in white willow that is extremely good for your heart. It can even be used as a medicine for heart attack and can save your life when you are out in the wild.

Chapter 2. Essential Oils for Pain relief

When you know that essential oils can be used in order to relieve pain in any part of human body. whereas, a question arises here that how one can use oils for the sake of pain relief. One of the best methods for using the essential oil is in the form of massage oils. Essential oils are highly concentrated and potent; therefore, such oils must be diluted with carrier oils like castor oil, olive oil, jojoba oil, coconut oil, sesame oil, sweet almond, avocado, apricot kernel etc.

A skin patch test is always recommended for all essential oils. This test patch can keep you safe from major harmful effects. It is better to apply the diluted form of oil on the forearm. Then keep an eye on the area that whether you are feeling pain or irritation for next 24 hours or not. if you are not feeling any kind of irritation for next 24 hours then it shows that the essential oil is right for you. You can prolong its use.

The number of drops that can be added to the carrier oils varies from one oil to another. one can add two different kinds of essential oils in order to maximize the effect of the oil. The one of the important thing that you must have to keep in your mind is that make sure that the oil is pure. If the essential oil will not be pure then it will not be as beneficial as much you thought.

Essential oils are considered as one of the best addition to the pain management program. When a person uses essential oil then it will reduce the usage of medicines for the sake of pain relief. When essential oils are used in bath creams and lotions, then it will increase the chances of pain relieving and relaxing in terms of massage therapy. There are various essential oils on the market that are popular for pain relief and relaxation. Usage of the essential oil varies from one type of pain to another.

Benefits of Essential Oils

Following are some of the significant benefits of essential oils.

- In order to fight flu and cough symptoms
- For relaxing the body and for soothing the sore muscles of the body
- It is also helpful in healing skin conditions
- Essential oils can also alleviate pain
- It is better in order to improve digestion
- Essential oils are considered as one of the best remedies for eliminating wrinkles and reducing cellulite
- One can also use essential oil for balancing the hormones
- It is used in almost all the homemade products for skin, beauty and health issues
-

Essential Oil Applications

Following are the four common ways through which essential oils can be used.

- Topical: One can use essential oils in a topical manner due to the easy penetration of oils in the cells and blood of the body. The essential oils move to all parts of the body with the help of blood and cells.
- Aromatic: As essential oils have a strong aroma; therefore, these are used in aromatherapy. When a person inhales the essential oils, it is absorbed into the bloodstream.
- Ingestion: Most of the essential oils are safe for internal use but make sure that it does not have highly powerful effects.
- Personal Care: It can be added in the homemade products and that product can be used for a number of reasons.

Safety rules and Preparations

Being the most concentrated form of the plant, it is also prone to being volatile, but not in the sense it will blow up in your face.

Simple rules

☐ Always wear gloves when mixing essential oils and making blends. This will make sure you don't suffer from contact dermatitis.

☐ Keep any and all essential oils out of the reach of the little ones. and pets.

☐ Store them in a dark and cool place. They will evaporate, even in the bottle, if exposed to high temperatures.

☐ NEVER use essential oils undiluted. There are websites out there that will tell you it's alright to do so. It's not.

Do a Patch test

Every skin reacts to essential oils differently. Some sensitive skins will form a rash or blisters. This is what is known as contact dermatitis. Doing a patch test will help you determine if you can use the oil or skip it. Your local health food store or herb shop can walk you through how to do a patch test.

Chapter 3. Pain Relief Remedies with Essential Oils

Following are some of the essential oils that can be used for reducing inflammation and pain. Take a look and rather than using any of the medicine for pain relief. Most of the essential oils are commonly available in the market. You can add up one or two essential oils together in order to increase the effects of the essential oils.

1. Chamomile oil

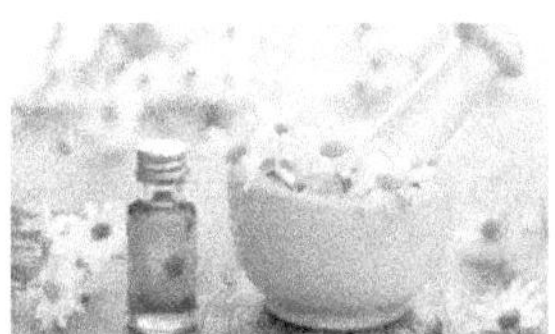

Chamomile oil is full of analgesic properties in order to soothe the pain in the inflamed muscles and joints. It can also be used for headaches, nerve pain and sore muscles like slipped discs and sciatica. Chamomile has soothing effect on the digestive system and can help in relieving pain caused by stomach cramping and excess gas. While looking at the method through which you can use chamomile oil in order to reduce the body pains is by adding few drops of it with carrier oil.

• You can add few drops of chamomile oil with coconut oil or sweet almond oil. Massage this oil on the painful joint or sore muscle.

• You can also add few drops of chamomile oil to diffuser. Inhale these therapeutic vapors deeply for almost 15 minutes. This inhaling will help you out in treating headache or migraine pains in couple of minutes.
You will feel good by performing either of the solution.

2. *Lavender oil*

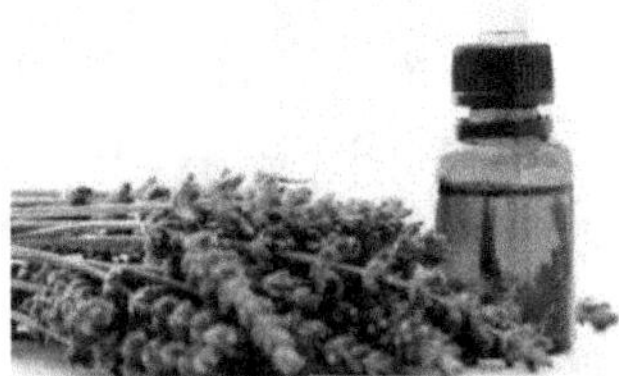

Lavender is one of the famous essential oil in order to treat pain in the joints and muscles. Lavender is used for centuries in order to treat pain in natural manner. lavender also acts like a mild sedative that can reduce anxiety and stress in quick manner. therefore, one can use lavender oil in order to get rid of headache due to tension. It is also considered as highly effective for muscles pain. Researches showed that lavender is full of anti-inflammatory as well as analgesic properties. When it comes to the method by which one can use lavender oil then its application as well as inhaling, both the methods are highly effective.

• For using lavender oil, you can add few drops of it to the diffuser. Inhale therapeutic vapors of lavender oil for almost 15 minutes. Your headache will go away completely as well as migraine.

• You can also apply lavender oil directly on the area where you are feeling pain. As lavender oil is mild therefore there is no need to add any carrier oil in it.

• Alternatively, pour two or three drops of lavender oil on your hand palms. Cup it over your nose and then take 3-5 slow and deep breaths. It will help you to fight against migraine.

• You can also add 2-5 drops of lavender essential oil on a cotton bud. Secure this cotton bud in zip lock bag. You can inhale this cotton bud whenever you are feeling headache.

3. Sweet marjoram essential oil

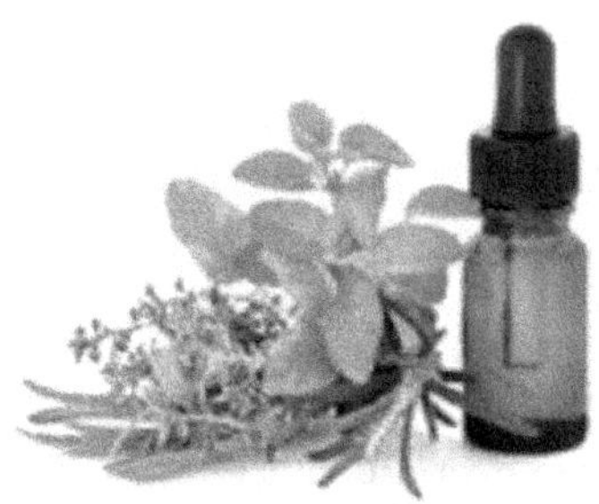

Sweet marjoram is such essential oil which is full of anti-inflammatory and sedative properties for reducing many types of pain in different body parts. It is considered as one of the effective solution for headache, nerve pain, migraines, stomach pains and other such kind of pain.

• You can use marjoram oil by adding it to black pepper oil, lavender oil and peppermint oil. Apply this mixture for four weeks and you will feel significant difference in the pain. This mixture is effective even for such pains that are for years and nothing is helpful in treating it.

• Marjoram oil is very helpful in treating toothache. Therefore, you can apply it directly on your tooth. While one can also add it to the toothpaste and then use it on your teeth.

4. Eucalyptus essential oil

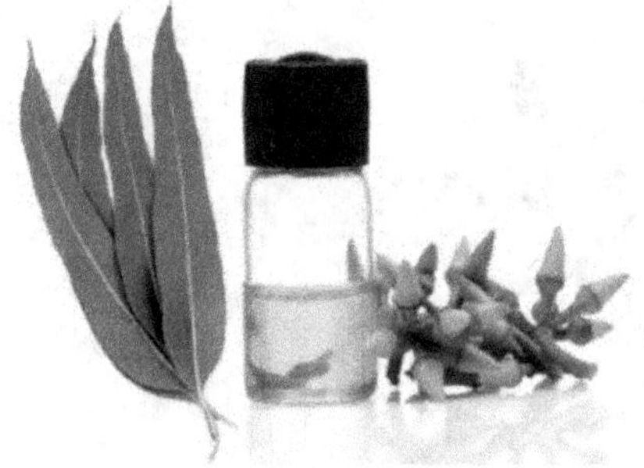

Eucalyptus essential oil is considered as one of the efficient pain reliever. This essential oil can be used in order to deal with nerve related issues as well as to get rid of the pain due to blocked sinuses. Even a few drops of eucalyptus oil are highly effective for headaches, arthritis, joint and muscles pains. Studies showed that eucalyptus oil is full of anti-inflammatory, antibacterial and antioxidant compounds.

• Add few drops of eucalyptus oil in diffuser and inhale it for 10 minutes. This inhaling is highly effective for post-surgery pain.

• You can apply eucalyptus oil on your joints and muscles by adding few drops of it in carrier oil. A little massage with eucalyptus oil is highly effective in order to cure body pains.

• Eucalyptus is also powerful essential oil for curing toothache. You can apply the oil directly on it or can add few drops of oil in your toothpaste. No matter how severe pain is, eucalyptus oil can treat it.

5. Peppermint essential oil

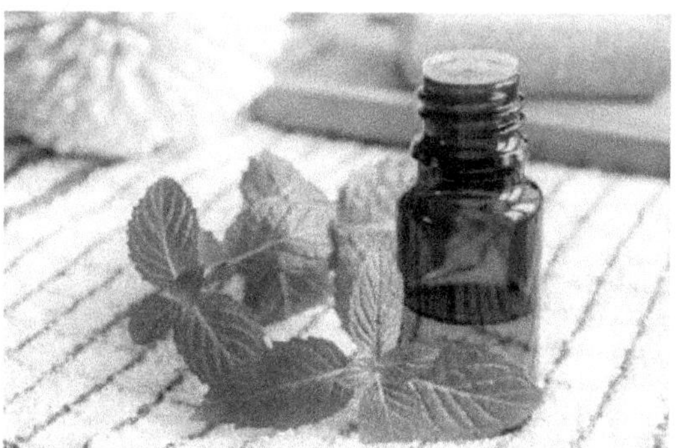

Peppermint essential oil is highly effective for the sake of treating intestinal and arthritis problems. Peppermint essential oil is full of anti-inflammatory, kills and deal with infections and antimicrobial.

It is also known as natural decongestant that can help you in dealing with blocked sinuses. There is high amount of menthol in it that make peppermint oil refreshing and cooling. Therefore, the cooling effect of the peppermint oil is helpful in releasing stress and tension.

• When you are feeling headache, one can directly apply peppermint oil on the forehead and massage for almost ten minutes.

• Due to the antispasmodic properties of the peppermint essential oil, one can use peppermint oil capsules in order to cure intestinal problems. It is considered as a safe and effective treatment of intestinal pains.

6. *Rosemary essential oil*

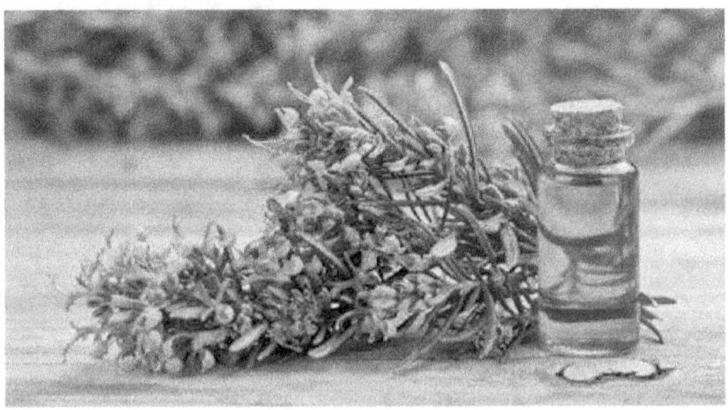

Rosemary oil is famous for its anti-inflammatory and analgesic properties and highly effective for chronic pain. This essential oil is also considered helpful in improving the circulation of blood in your body and for relieving muscles spasm. It is used in most of the pain relief medications due to its properties of reducing pain and inflammation.

• You can use rosemary oil for pain relief by adding few drops of this oil in any of the carrier oil and apply directly on the painful area.

• One can also add drops of the oil in lotions or creams and then apply it on the affected area for 10 minutes.

• Mixing rosemary oil with any other essential oil can also be effective for pain relief.

7. Thyme essential oil

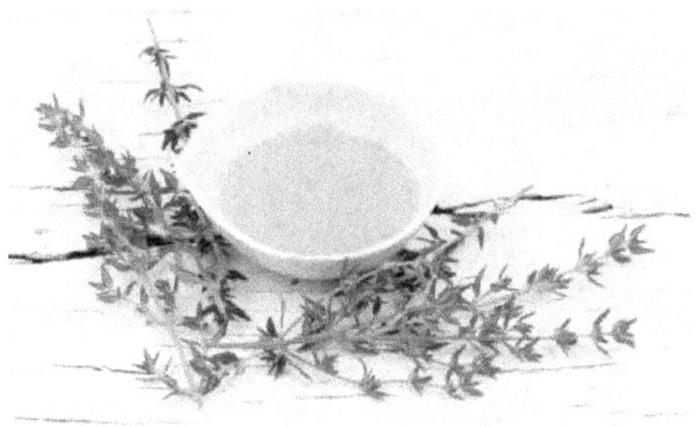

Thyme essential oil can be used in order to treat muscles pains, inflammation in joints or backache. It can also be helpful in dealing with acute as well as chronic pain. Thyme is full of anti-inflammatory properties that make it easy to penetrate inside the skin and body of the person in order to relief pain. You can also use this oil in order to cure various diseases.

• One can use thyme oil by adding few drops of it in any carrier oil and then apply the oil on the affected area.

• You can also pour few drops of thyme oil in your diffuser for the sake of inhaling it. inhale this mixture for almost 10-15 minutes and you will feel much better. It is highly helpful in treating headache due to the cool and refreshing aroma of the thyme oil.

• It is also perfect for aromatherapy due to its strong and healing aroma.

8. *Clary sage essential oil*

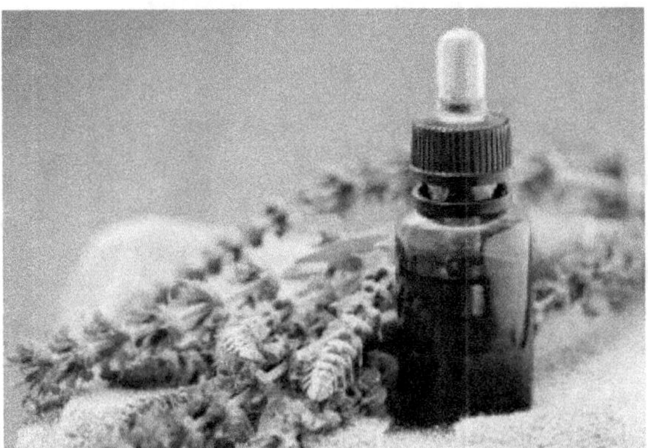

It is also known as Salvia sclarea, essential oil is also very powerful pain reliever. It is considered highly effective in dealing with menstrual pains and muscles cramps. Due to the analgesic effect of this essential oil make it highly effective.

• For menstrual pain, one can add Salvia sclarea oil in lavender and rose oil. Massage this oil daily on your abdominal area. one will feel difference in menstrual pain after one or two days usage of this oil mixture. It can also be helpful for abdominal cramping.

• Due to the relaxant properties of clary sage, it has calming effect. one can apply this oil on the forehead in order to treat headache.

9. Sandalwood essential oil

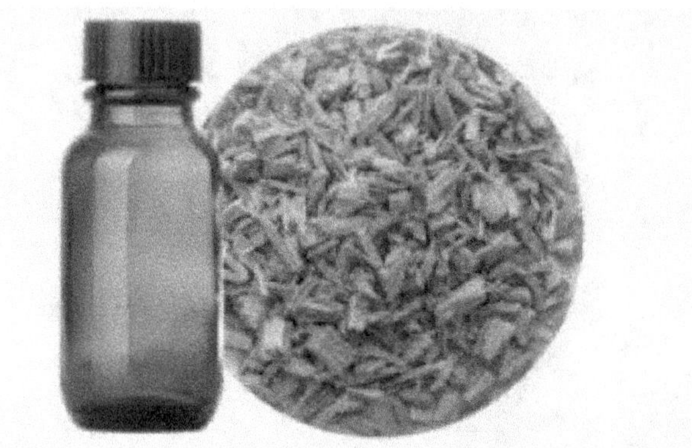

Sandalwood essential oil is very powerful oil in dealing with joint pain and muscles inflammation. It is also helpful in relaxing muscles and in order to prevent muscles spasms. It deals with the nerves pain by sedating your nervous system. The adrenaline production is reduced due to this essential oil.

• You can add sandalwood essential oil with carrier oil in order to make a painkilling ointment for knee pain, rheumatic conditions and sore muscles.

• You can also add this essential oil in diffuser and then inhale the oil for almost 10-15 minutes. The cooling and soothing aroma of the essential oil will treat headache and migraine. You will feel better after half an hour after the application of this essential oil.

10. Juniper essential oil

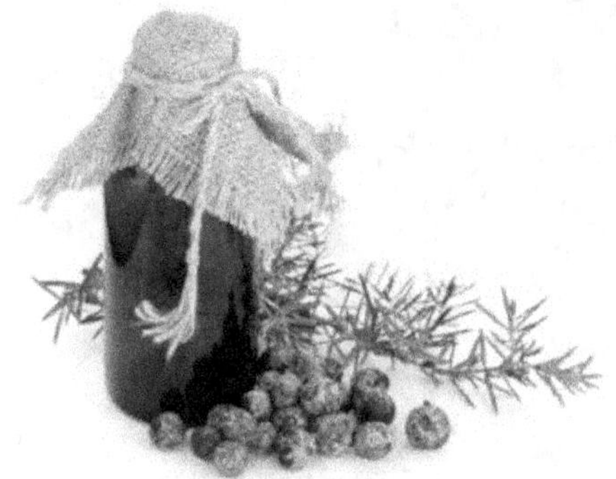

Juniper essential oil is a perfect way in order to deal with muscles pain and stiffness related to the arthritis, gout and rheumatism. It is also helpful to reduce pain and to treat painful joints as well as painful muscles.

• One can add few drops of juniper essential oil with any of the carrier oil in order to make pain relief ointment. You can apply the oil directly on the body part where one is feeling pain.

• One can also add few drops of juniper essential oil in to a bath and soak your body in it for half an hour. This soaking will help you in dealing with the muscles pain.

11. *Ginger essential oil*

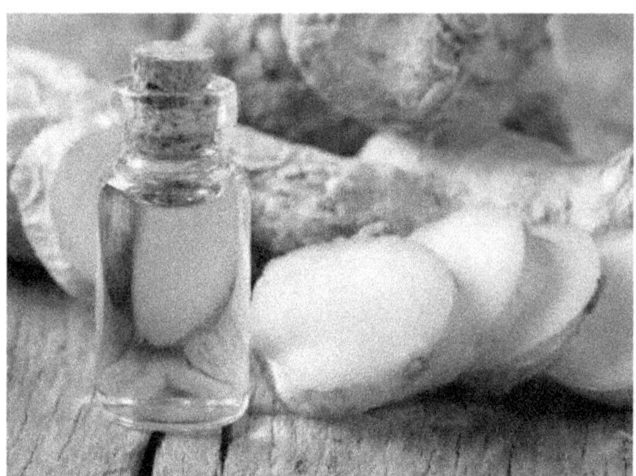

Ginger essential oil is perfect solution in order to alleviate muscles pain and to ease stiffness. There is a compound in ginger that is known as gingerol that contains anti-inflammatory and analgesic properties. When you massage ginger oil on painful muscles or sore joints, you can relieve the pain. Ginger oil is considered as an effective natural remedy in order to deal with joint inflammation, menstrual cramps, osteoarthritis and rheumatoid arthritis. Ginger essential oil is full of pain relieving effect like present in ibuprofen.

• You can use ginger oil on painful joints and muscles by adding few drops of oil in any of the carrier oil. Massage this oil for 10 minutes on the painful area. You will feel significant difference in the pain.

• Ginger essential oil can also be used in aromatherapy in order to release tension, stress and to treat headache.

12. Frankincense essential oil

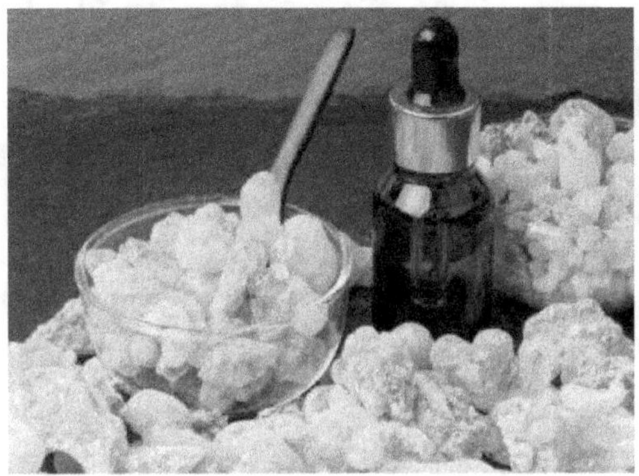

Frankincense essential oil is known for its anti-inflammatory as well as analgesic properties. It is also effective in reducing muscles tension as it helps in reducing stress and relaxing your muscles. This essential oil is full of pain-relieving properties that make it perfect home remedy in order to get rid of pain. It is considered highly effective in blocking COX-2.

• If you want to use Frankincense essential oil for pain reduction, then add few drops of this essential oil in any of the carrier oil. Apply this mixture on the affected area and massage for 5 minutes. You will feel difference in intensity of pain.

• You can also add this essential oil in diffuser. Inhale it for around 10-15 minutes and you will feel better. It is very powerful in releasing stress and tension that leads to treatment of headache.

• You can also add Frankincense essential oil along with other essential oils like ginger, thyme etc. in order to increase the effect of this oil and to get better results.

13. Yarrow essential oil

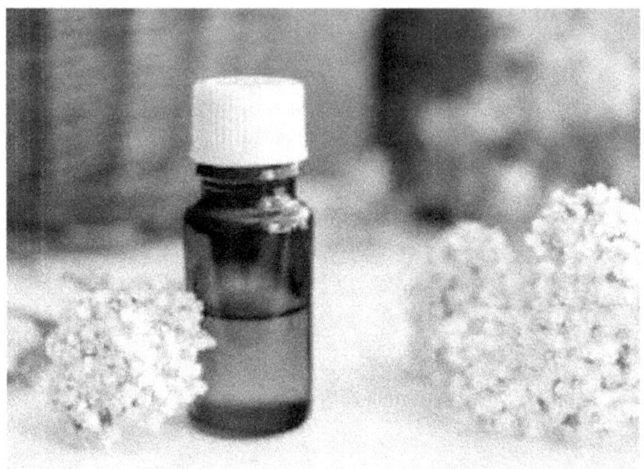

Yarrow essential oil is very famous due to its medicinal properties. This oil is considered as one of the best method to deal with rheumatic pain and intestinal cramping. Many people make teas using yarrow herb in order to treat abdominal pain and inflammation as well as the gastric issues.

• As this essential oil has mild effects, therefore you can apply the oil directly on the painful joint or sore muscle. This oil will quickly work in reducing the pain.

• You can also add other essential oils along with this essential oil in order to enhance the properties of this oil. Then apply the oil on the painful area and you will feel the difference.

14. Wintergreen essential oil

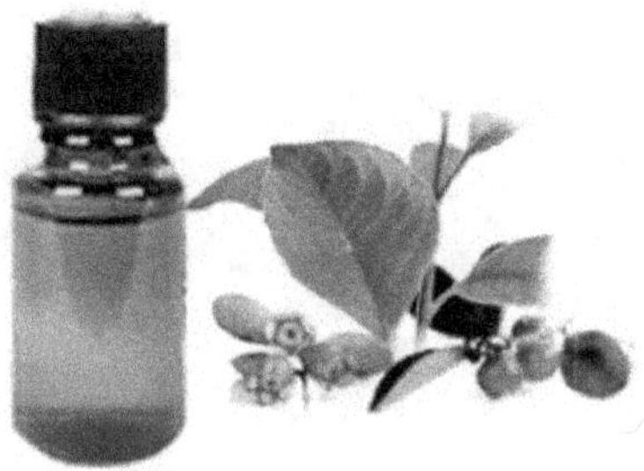

Wintergreen essential oil is one of the most effective solution in order to deal with muscles aches, lower back pain, and stiff joints. This essential oil is similar to aspirin in terms of pain management. One of the benefit of this oil is that it does not have any side effects and help you in releasing the pain without harming your body.

• You can add few drops of Wintergreen essential oil along with any of the carrier oil. Massage this oil on the affected area. you will feel difference in few minutes.

• This essential oil can also be added in painkiller creams and lotion. Apply these creams and lotions on your affected areas and you will feel better as well as significant reduction in pain.

15. Vetiver

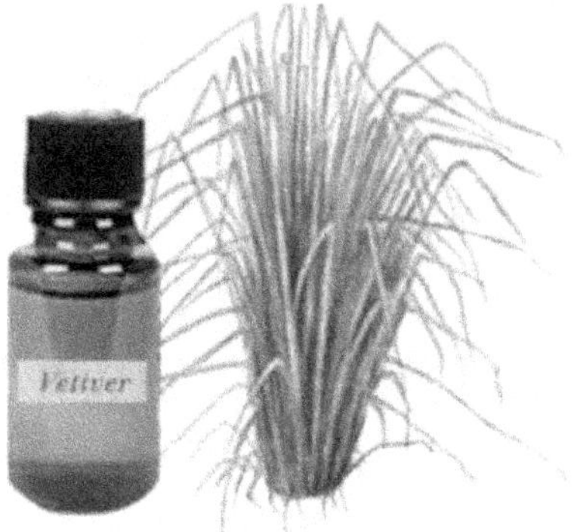

Vetiver is also very helpful in terms of dealing with the pain. Although this herb is not famous in most of the countries as it is not easily available in all the areas. The antiinflammation properties of the essential oil provide relief to your nervous and circulatory system. You can use this oil in order to deal with general pains and aches like rheumatism, muscular pain, arthritis and headache.

• You can use this oil directly on your skin in order to deal with stress, muscles pain and joint pain.

Tips to Choose Right Essential Oils and Herbs

1. How to Choose High—Quality Essential Oils:

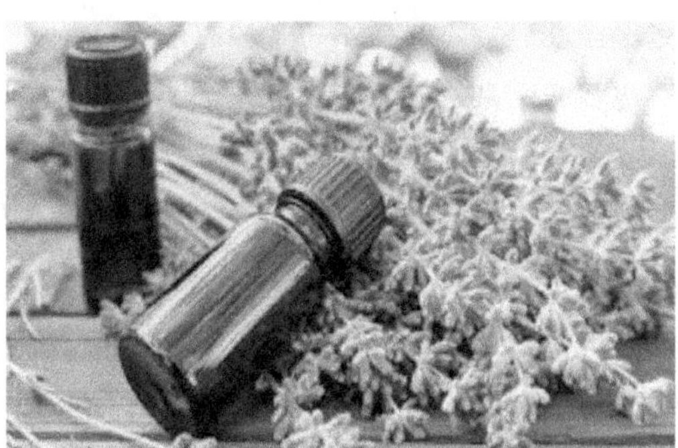

Essential Oil Testing

There must be the botanical or scientific name of each plant on the bottle. There should be the description of the expiry date, the process of extraction of oil, and origin of the plant.

Unsprayed, Wild Crafted, or Organic

First of all, seek for those oils that are organic. There might be the concentration of the pollutants in the essential oil. It is true in case of citrus essential oils because pesticides are excessively sprayed on them. By the word organic, we mean different things are found in different continents, and it is a sign of quality. Some of the sellers have those oils that are unsprayed. There are various higher quality oils which are wild crafted too.

Variety of Products Offered

There are many varieties of aromatherapy essential oils. Many retailers sell different essential oils. So, it is not necessary that you will find the same essential oils from some other retailer. You need to check the ingredients on the packaging of the oil. Buy the essential oil from that retailer whose oil has same ingredients that you are looking for. So, in this way, you will not get the essential oil that contains some other ingredients that you do not need.

What to Look for in Essential Oils

Label: Check out the label carefully. It must have an expiry date, country of origin, plant part, Botanical name, chemotype, and distillation date. You also see "Keep Out of Reach of Children" statement. This statement should be there on the label. Cost: See the cost of the essential oil on its label.

Chapter 4. Effective Natural Remedies to Relieve Pain with herbs

1. Turmeric & Ginger

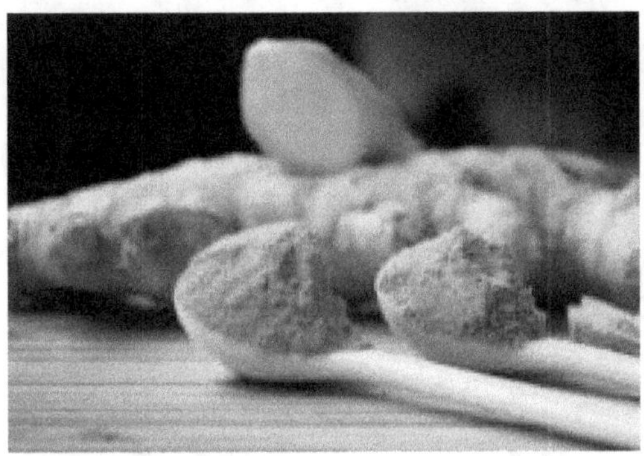

Ingredients:

- Fresh ginger – ½ teaspoon
- Turmeric root (powdered) – ½ teaspoon
- Honey – as required

Directions:

➢ Blend 1/2 teaspoon of powder of turmeric root and fresh ginger.

➢ Pour 2 cups of water, turmeric powder, and ginger in a pan for 10 to 15 minutes.

➢ Then strain the herbs out and sweeten the tea with honey and take it daily.

2. Blackstrap Molasses

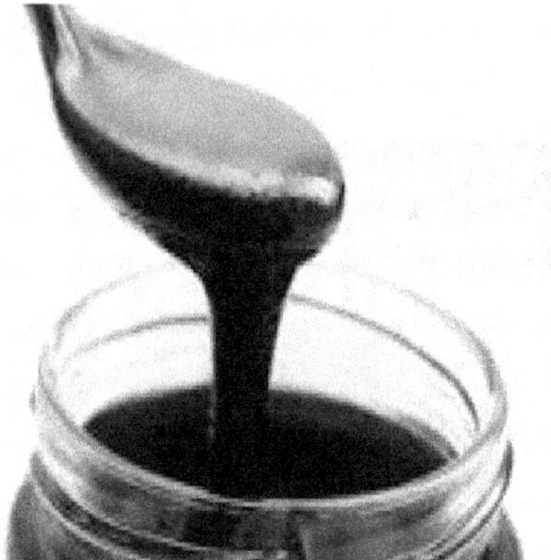

Ingredients:

- Water - 1 cup
- Blackstrap molasses – 1 tablespoon

Directions:

➢ Heat a pan on medium heat and pour 1 cup of water until warm but not hot.

➢ Put in 1 tablespoon of blackstrap molasses and drink one cup of tea daily.

➢ You will permanently get rid of joint pain.

3. Willow Bark (Salicin)

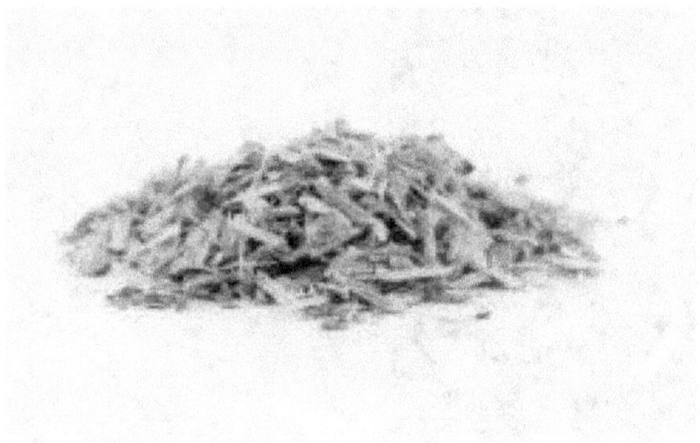

Ingredients:

- Dried willow bark - 1 tablespoon
- Fresh water – 1 cup
- Honey – as required

Directions:

➢   Take a pan and pour 1cup of water into it. Now, put 1 tablespoon of dried willow bark for 10 to 15 minutes.

➢   Just like numerous herbal teas, willow bark tea is also bitter. You can add honey to make it sweet.

➢   Take willow bark tea 2 times a day to get rid of joint pain.

4. Capsaicin Hot Pepper Cream

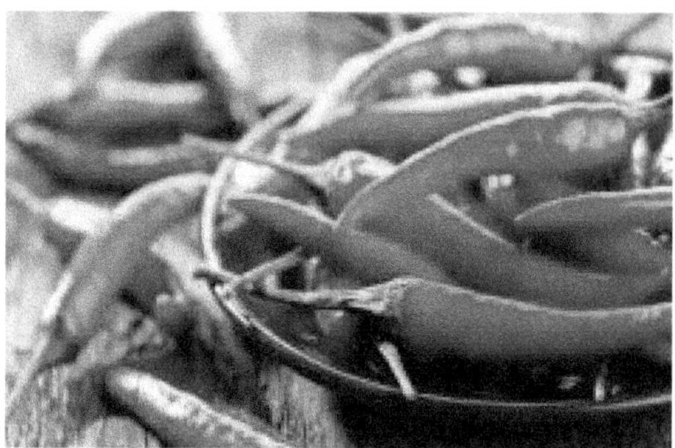

Ingredients:

- Cayenne powder - 3 tablespoons
- Grape seed oil - 1 cup
- Grated beeswax - 1/2 cup
- Double boiler - 1
- A jar with a tight lid

Directions:

➢ Combine 3 tablespoons of cayenne powder and 1 cup of grape seed oil or any other oil of your own choice. For 5 to 10 minutes, heat them in a double boiler.

➢ Pour 1/2 cup beeswax. Stir it until gets melted thoroughly. Cook it until every ingredient is mixed well.

➤	Put this in the refrigerator and allow the mixture to cool. Again mix it well.

➤	Again chill it for 15 more minutes and mix it once again before putting this mixture in a jar. Cover it with a tight lid and refrigerate it.

➤	You can keep it for 1 ½ weeks. Apply daily to get rid of joint pain.

5. Juniper Berry

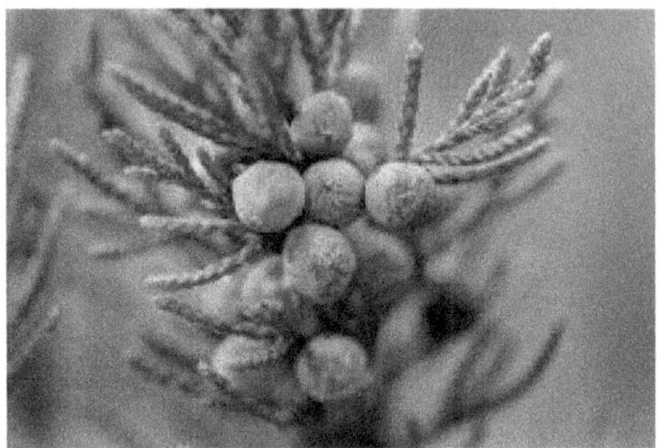

Ingredients:

- Fresh water - 1 cup
- Dried juniper berries - 1 tablespoon
- Honey - as required

Directions:

➢ Take a pan and heat it on medium heat.

➢ Boil 1 cup water.

➢ Take a cup and put 1 tablespoon juniper berries in it.

➢ Now, pour hot water in the cup and leave for 20 minutes and sieve it.

➢ Take 1 cup two times a day. Put honey in the tea if you want to sweeten it up.

6. Pectin

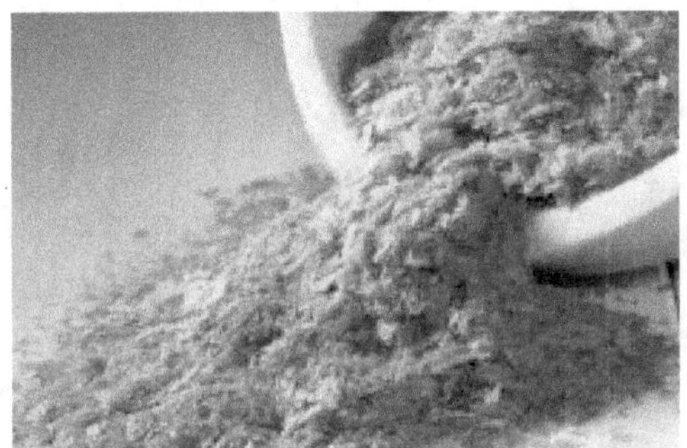

Ingredients:

- Liquid pectin - 1 tablespoon
- Grape juice - 8 oz.

Directions:

➢ Combine 1 tablespoon pectin and 8 oz. grape juice. Drink it twice daily.

➢ This might take almost 2 weeks to see its results.

➢ It is more reliable in results than pain relievers.

7. Burdock Root

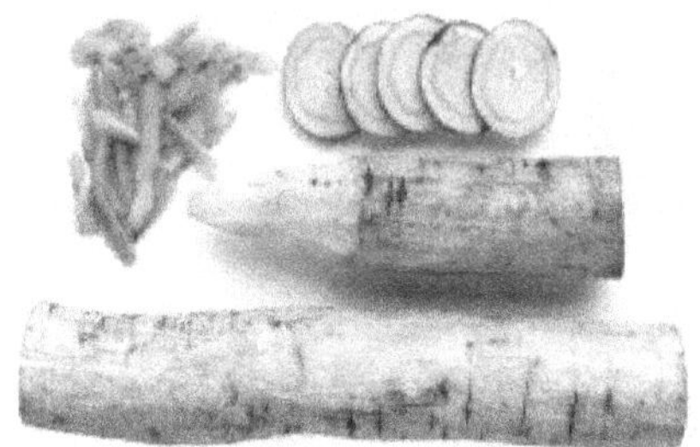

Ingredients:

- Dried burdock root - 1 tablespoon
- Fresh water - 1 cup

Directions:

- Heat a pan with 1 cup of water over medium heat.

- Put 1 tablespoon of burdock root into the hot water.

- Heat for 15 minutes and sieve it.

- Drink this tea 4 times a day and. You will get rid of joint pain.

8. Fenugreek Seeds

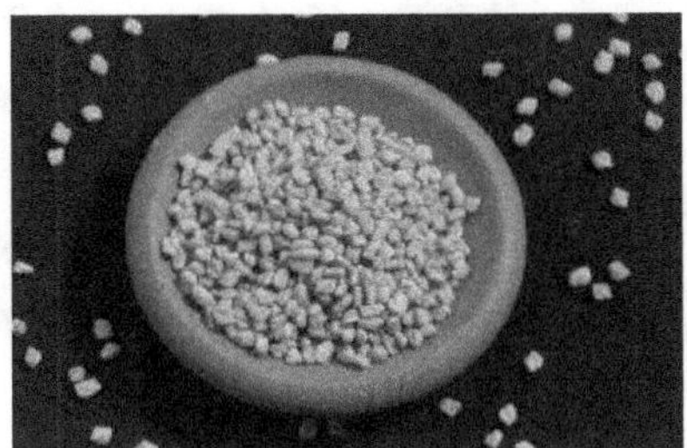

Fenugreek seeds are not very much desired and well-liked than a few of other herbs. But the fact is that this herb has very strong cardio-protective advantages because it is enriched with antioxidants. It is very helpful in preventing the obesity problem by controlling sugar level of blood.

Ingredients:

- Fenugreek seeds - 1 teaspoon
- Fresh water - 1 cup

Directions:

➢ Pour 1 teaspoon of fenugreek seeds in 1 cup of fresh water for the whole night.

➢ In the morning, sieve out the fenugreek seeds from the water. Eat these soaked fenugreek seeds on a clear stomach.

➢ Follow this remedy on a daily basis for the best results.

9.Naturally Healthy

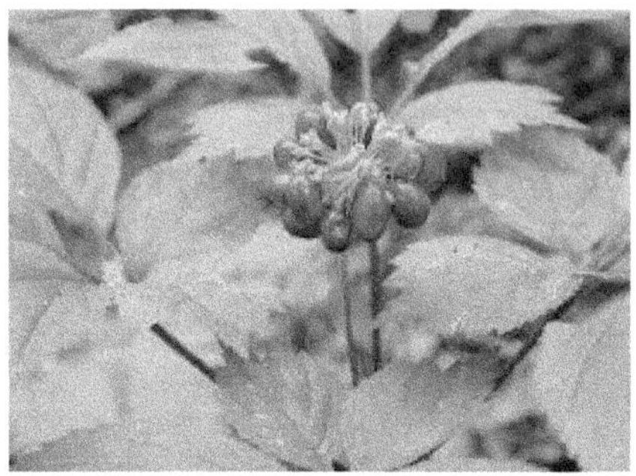

Ingredients:

- 1 teaspoon kava kava
- 1 teaspoon dried devil's claw
- 1 teaspoon dried ginseng

Directions:

For tea:

➢ Crush the herbs and roll in a paper towel, then place them in your tea ball. If you are using powdered herbs, the paper towel is important to allow the flavor out without your cup being filled with the powder. For taste, you can add 1 tablespoon honey or 2 packets of stevia.

➢ Drink up to 2 cups per day, or blend it in a smoothie with fruit (up to 2 cups per day.)

For Salve:

➢   Crush the herbs as small as you can get them, then mix with either your favorite unscented lotion or petroleum jelly. Apply to affected area, removing with a warm washcloth after 20 minutes.

➢   Repeat morning and night, or as often as needed for maximum comfort.

10. Like New

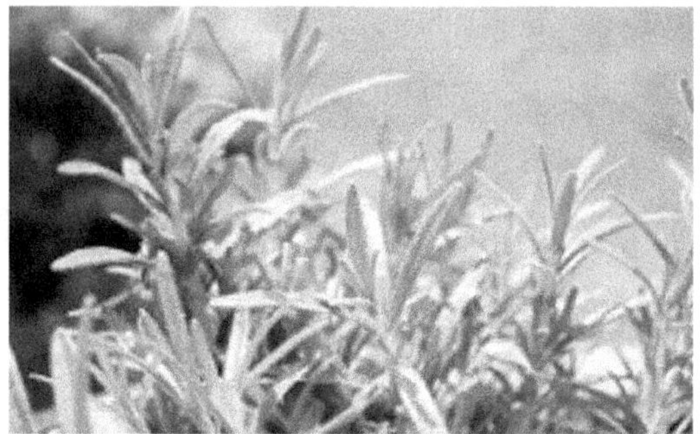

Ingredients:

- 1 teaspoon dried rose hips
- 1 teaspoon dried lavender leaves
- 1 teaspoon dried capsaicin

Directions:

For tea:

➢ Crush the herbs and roll in a paper towel, then place them in your tea ball. If you are using powdered herbs, the paper towel is important to allow the flavor out without your cup being filled with the powder. For taste, you can add 1 tablespoon honey or 2 packets of stevia.

➢ Drink up to 2 cups per day, or blend it in a smoothie with fruit (up to 2 cups per day.)

For Salve:

➢	Crush the herbs as small as you can get them, then mix with either your favorite unscented lotion or petroleum jelly. Apply to affected area, removing with a warm washcloth after 20 minutes.

➢	Repeat morning and night, or as often as needed for maximum comfort.

11. Rejuvenation Station

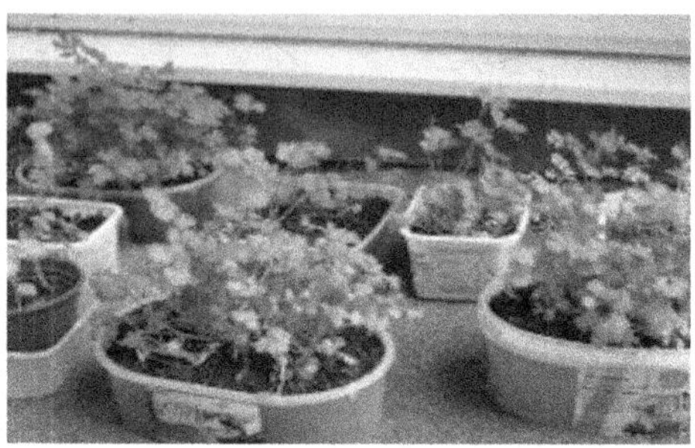

Ingredients:

- 1 teaspoon dried licorice leaves
- 1 teaspoon fennel seeds
- 1 teaspoon dried marjoram

Directions:

For tea:

➢ Crush the herbs and roll in a paper towel, then place them in your tea ball. If you are using powdered herbs, the paper towel is important to allow the flavor out without your cup being filled with the powder. For taste, you can add 1 tablespoon honey or 2 packets of stevia.

➢ Drink up to 2 cups per day, or blend it in a smoothie with fruit (up to 2 cups per day.)

For Salve:

> ➢ Crush the herbs as small as you can get them, then mix with either your favorite unscented lotion or petroleum jelly. Apply to affected area, removing with a warm washcloth after 20 minutes.

> ➢ Repeat morning and night, or as often as needed for maximum comfort.

12.Better Than Drugs

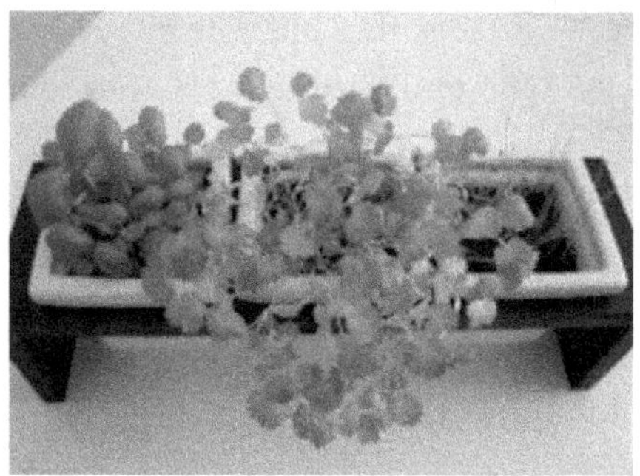

Ingredients:

- 1 teaspoon cayenne
- 1 teaspoon black pepper
- 1 teaspoon turmeric
- 1 teaspoon dried ginseng

Directions:

For tea:

➢ Crush the herbs and roll in a paper towel, then place them in your tea ball. If you are using powdered herbs, the paper towel is important to allow the flavor out without your cup being filled with the powder. For taste, you can add 1 tablespoon honey or 2 packets of stevia.

➢ Drink up to 2 cups per day, or blend it in a smoothie with fruit (up to 2 cups per day.)

For Salve:

➤ Crush the herbs as small as you can get them, then mix with either your favorite unscented lotion or petroleum jelly. Apply to affected area, removing with a warm washcloth after 20 minutes.

➤ Repeat morning and night, or as often as needed for maximum comfort.

13.Herbal Healing

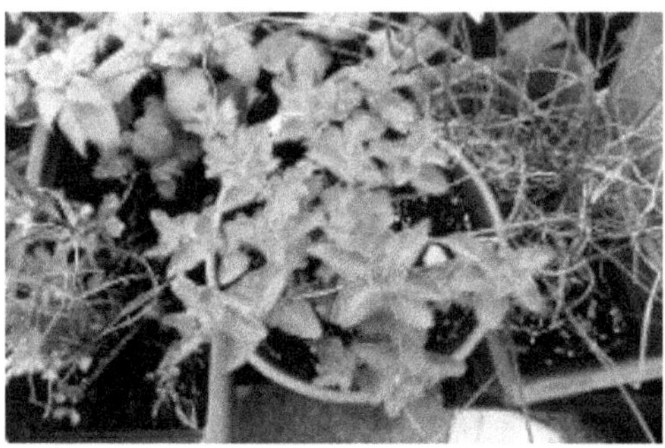

Ingredients:

- 1 teaspoon dried capsaicin
- 1 teaspoon dried St. John's Wort
- 1 teaspoon dried rose petals

Directions:

For tea:

➢ Crush the herbs and roll in a paper towel, then place them in your tea ball. If you are using powdered herbs, the paper towel is important to allow the flavor out without your cup being filled with the powder. For taste, you can add 1 tablespoon honey or 2 packets of stevia.

➢ Drink up to 2 cups per day, or blend it in a smoothie with fruit (up to 2 cups per day.)

For Salve:

➢	Crush the herbs as small as you can get them, then mix with either your favorite unscented lotion or petroleum jelly. Apply to affected area, removing with a warm washcloth after 20 minutes.

➢	Repeat morning and night, or as often as needed for maximum comfort.

14. It's all in the Leaves

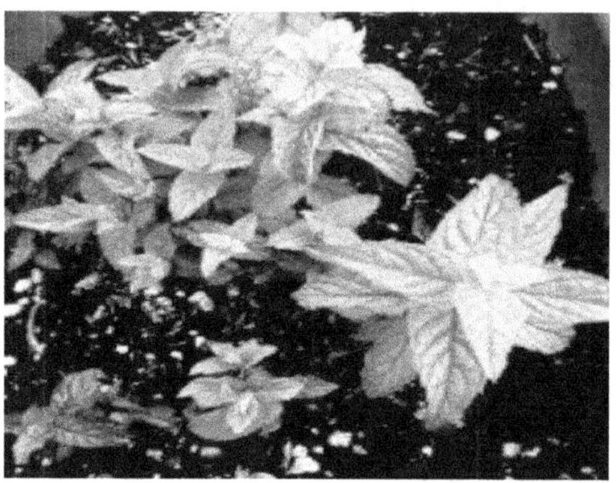

Ingredients:

- 1 teaspoon black tea leaves
- 1 teaspoon feverfew
- 1 teaspoon ginger

Directions:

For tea:

➤ Crush the herbs and roll in a paper towel, then place them in your tea ball. If you are using powdered herbs, the paper towel is important to allow the flavor out without your cup being filled with the powder. For taste, you can add 1 tablespoon honey or 2 packets of stevia.

➤ Drink up to 2 cups per day, or blend it in a smoothie with fruit (up to 2 cups per day.)

For Salve:

➢	Crush the herbs as small as you can get them, then mix with either your favorite unscented lotion or petroleum jelly. Apply to affected area, removing with a warm washcloth after 20 minutes.

➢	Repeat morning and night, or as often as needed for maximum comfort.

15. Tricky Tonic

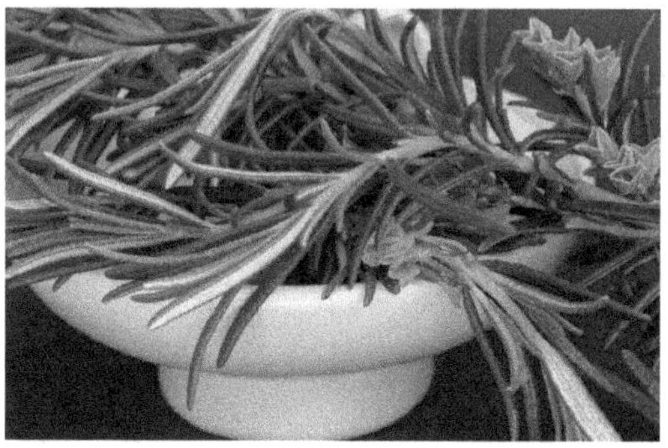

Ingredients:

- 1 teaspoon dried oregano
- 1 teaspoon dried rosemary leaves
- 1 teaspoon dried basil leaves

Directions:

For tea:

➢ Crush the herbs and roll in a paper towel, then place them in your tea ball. If you are using powdered herbs, the paper towel is important to allow the flavor out without your cup being filled with the powder. For taste, you can add 1 tablespoon honey or 2 packets of stevia.

➢ Drink up to 2 cups per day, or blend it in a smoothie with fruit (up to 2 cups per day.)

For Salve:

➤   Crush the herbs as small as you can get them, then mix with either your favorite unscented lotion or petroleum jelly. Apply to affected area, removing with a warm washcloth after 20 minutes.

➤   Repeat morning and night, or as often as needed for maximum comfort.

Fresh Herb Tips

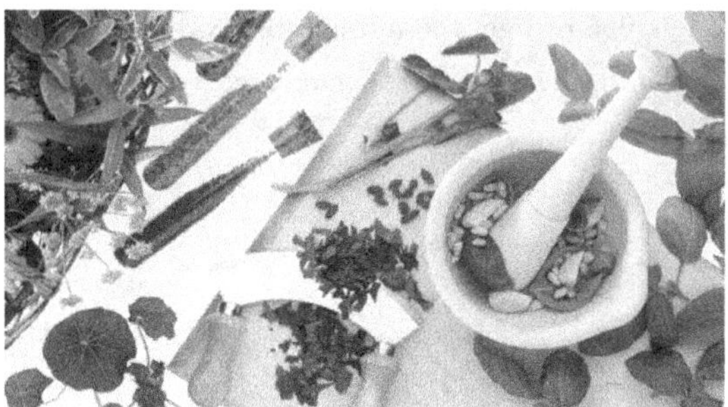

Be careful while cooking the herbs. If you put more herbs than needed, then its flavor will change. On the other hand, if you will put fewer herbs then it will be tasteless. Hence, initially put the little amount and then increase the amount of herbs. In this way, you will not make a mistake. The following tips will help you.

Tips:

Stand tall

Select those herbs that are straight. Herbs should be held vertically without falling. Leaves should be of fresh colors. There should be no brown spots on them. Their smell must be fresh.

Store away

You should refrigerate the herbs so that they can last for more days. If leaves are small or flat, you might put them in some wet paper towel and seal them in a bag. If you have many herbs, then put them vertically in a vase that must be full of water before putting them into the refrigerator.

The dry alternative

Dried herbs are not very useful as fresh herbs. So, always try to buy fresh herbs. Do not buy dried herbs. In case if you are using dried herbs then mix 1 teaspoon of dried herbs and 1 tablespoon of fresh herbs. Fresh herbs have more benefits than dried herbs.

Conclusion

A vast number of people around the globe use essential oils, botanical and herbal in order to attain natural methods of health care. With regard to the medicinal plants and herbs, the place is wider than a curative aspect only.

They often find a tighter and prominent space in the cultural fabric embedded within particular social groups. So you can see Medicinal herbs used as herbal baths, extracts, powders, teas, powders, salves, poultices, or syrups.

Any herbs can have medicinal benefits if there is the presence of some chemical components in the structure of the herb which can provoke a specific response within the human body. The specific dosage and its potency will significantly depend on the specific part of the herb utilized, the particular season on which it is grown, and even upon the specific composition of the soil used to grow the medicinal herb.

BONUS CHAPTER

Helichrysum essential oil

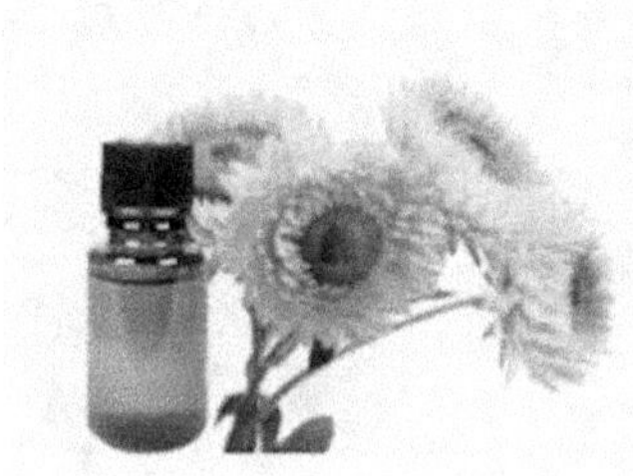

It is one of the most powerful essential oil that is highly effective in dealing with the damaged and dry skin. Helichrysum essential oil is full of anti-inflammatory as well as analgesic properties. One can reduce chronic and for nerve pain by using this essential oil. It can be used in order to treat burnt skin and to remove the sunburn marks from your face.

• Helichrysum essential oil can be directly applied to the area of injury in order to reduce pain and to pevent bruising.

• You can also add few drops of Helichrysum essential oil in any of the carrier oil. After adding both the oils, you can apply this mixture on any area where you are feeling pain. Massage the oil for almost 10 minutes and you will feel significant difference in your pain.

• It can also be added in face creams and lotions for removing the pigment, scars and to give you glowing skin.

Oregano essential oil

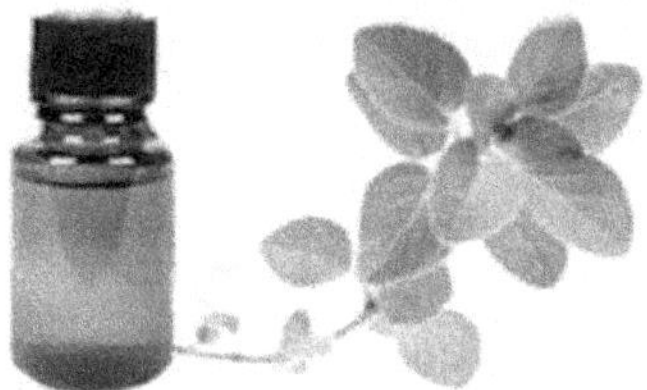

Oregano is one of the soothing essential oil that contains antioxidant properties in order to deal with pain and inflammation. From simple headache to fresh wounds to chronic pain, everything can be treated well by using oregano essential oil.

• You can add few drops of oregano essential oil along with any of the carrier oil in order to soothe pain.

• You can also add oregano essential oil in the diffuser and inhale it for almost 10-15 minutes in order to get rid of stress and tension for reliving headache.

St. John's Wort essential oil

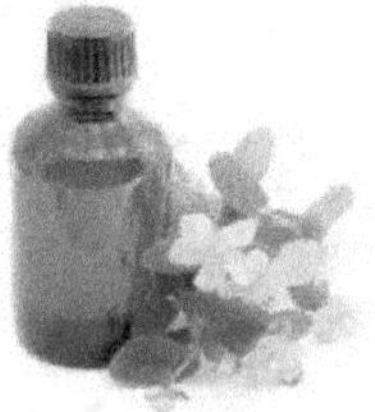

St. John's Wort essential oil is one of the powerful essential herb that is associated with mood and depression. You can use this oil in order to reduce pain in any part of your body. the soothing inflammation of this essential oil is often used as precursor to pain. It is one of the most effective herb for dealing with pain. St. John's Wort essential oil is easily available in the food stores as well as in natural herbs shops.

• You can use St. John's Wort essential herb by directly applying it on the affected area for almost one week.

• You can also add few drops of St. John's Wort essential oil in any of the carrier oil. Apply this mixture on the painful muscles and massage for 10 minutes. After 10 minutes, you will feel significant difference in the pain. Continue the usage of the essential oil for almost a week.

• You can also add St. John's Wort essential oil in a diffuser. Inhale the diffuser for 10 minutes and repeat it throughout the day. The soothing aroma of the essential oil will help you in releasing tension and in soothing your nerves resulting in pain relief.

Devil's Claw essential oil

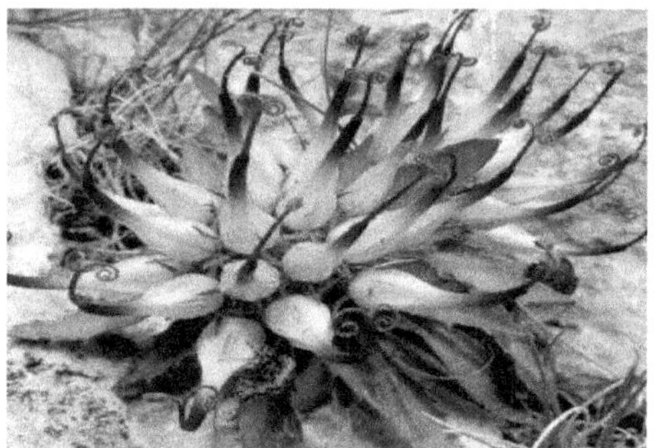

Devil's Claw is one of the oldest essential herb that is used as pain relieving medication. The soothing effect of this essential oil can relieve pain in almost all part of the body. the potential effects of Devil's Claw essential oil help in eliminating arthritis pain. There are wide range of unique compounds in devil's claw like harpagoside and other analgesic compounds. These compounds make it easy for you to deal with pain any part of the body.

• One can use Devil's Claw essential oil topically by applying it on the affected body part.

• You can also add few drops of this essential oil with any of the carrier oil for pain relief

• The refreshing aroma of Devil's Claw essential oil make it perfect for adding to your diffuser and then inhale it in order to get relief from pain like headache.

Turmeric essential oil

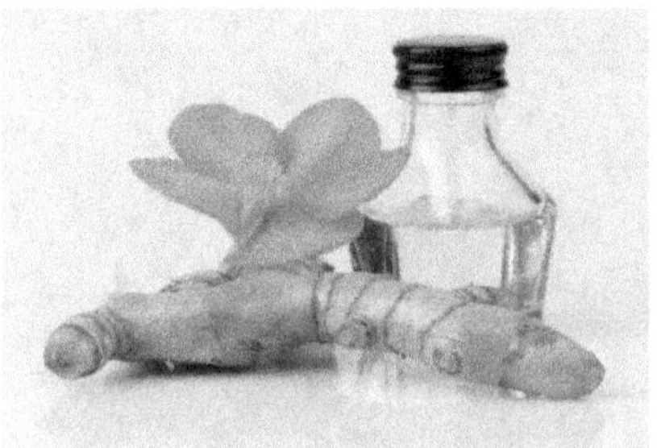

Turmeric is considered as one of best anti-inflammatory herbs for pain relief. It is helpful in reducing the strain on the immune system of a person. This essential oil inhibit communication between pain receptors and inflammatory triggers. This essential oil is helpful in dealing with acute as well as chronic pain.

• You can apply turmeric essential oil by adding few drops of it in carrier oil. Apply this oil on the painful muscle and massage for 10 minutes.

• One can also add turmeric essential oil along with other essential oils in order to enhance the overall properties of the oil.